COLORFUL PICTURE BOOK OF HYMNS

"Therefore I will give thanks to You,
among the nations, O Lord,
and I will sing praises to Your name."

Psalm 18:49

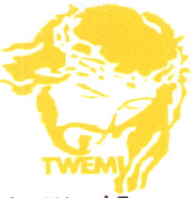

Copyright © 2020 The Word Evangelical Ministries Inc.
www.amazon.com/author/tweminc
All Rights Reserved.

Amazing Grace

Amazing Grace,

how sweet the sound,

That saved a wretch like me.

I once was lost,

but now am found,

Was blind, but now, I see.

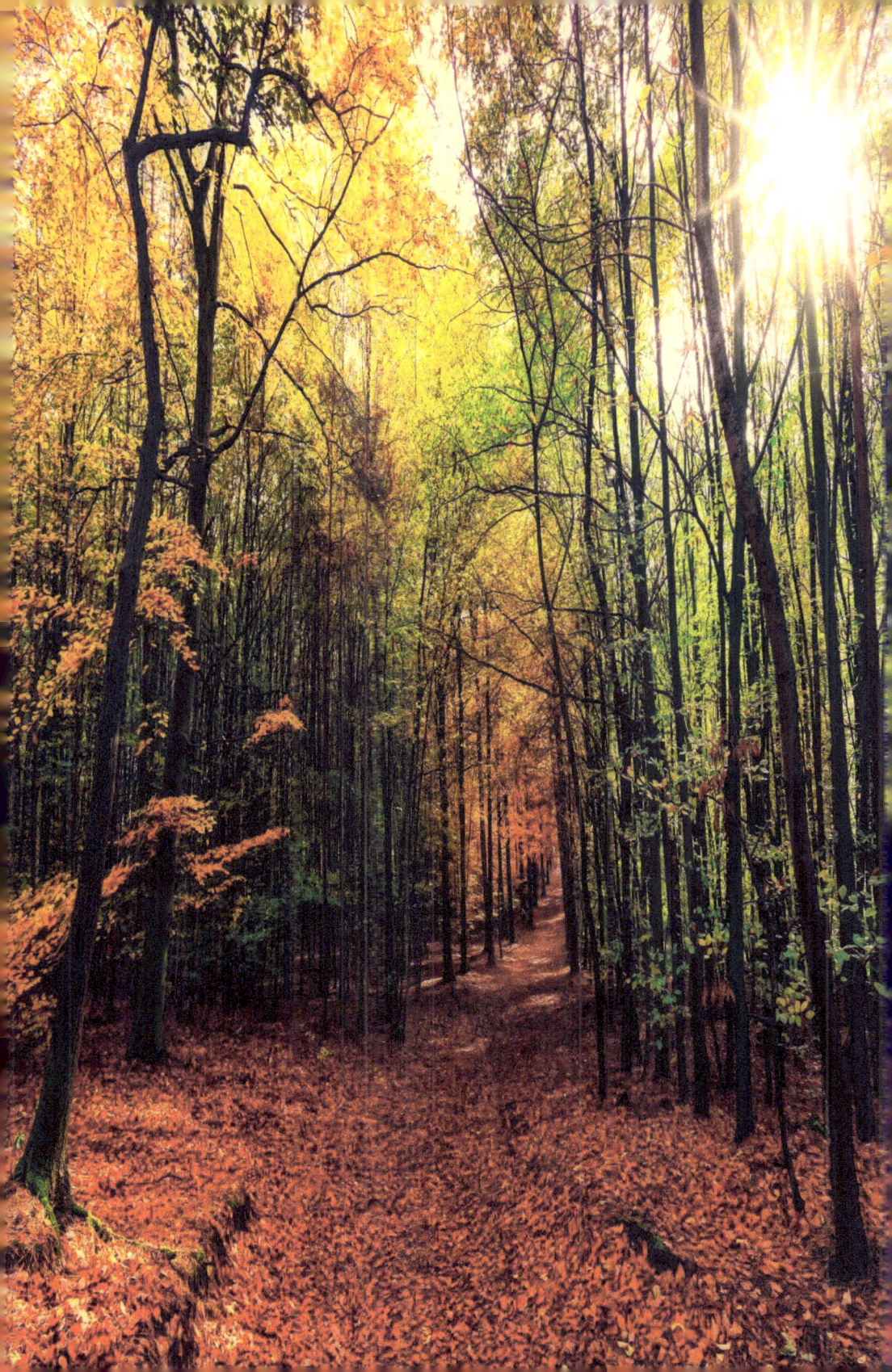

All Things Bright And Beautiful Hymn

All things bright and beautiful,

All creatures great and small,

All things wise and wonderful,

The Lord God made them all.

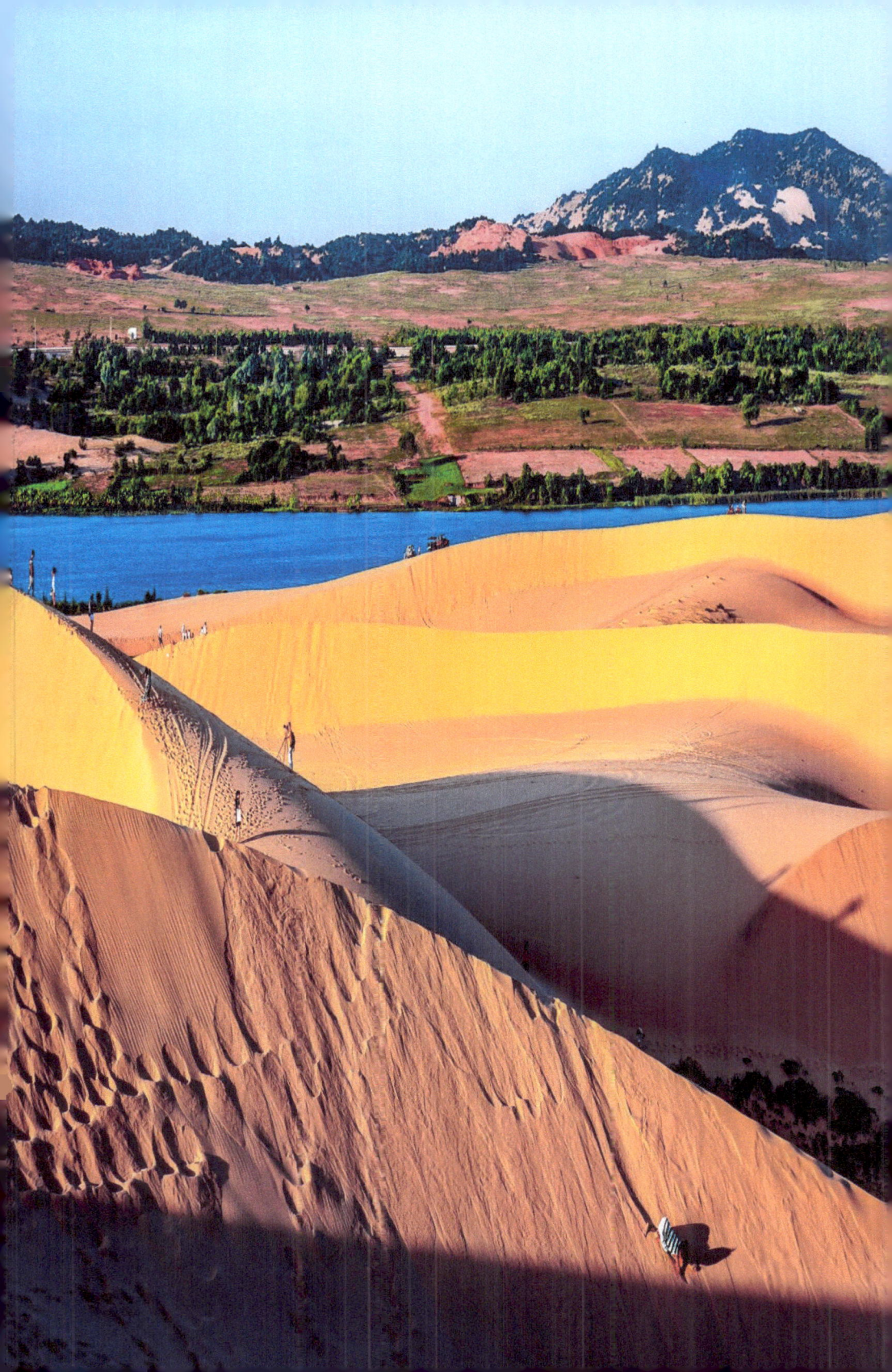

In the Garden

I come to the garden,

While the dew,

is still on the roses;

And the voice I hear,

falling on my ear,

Praise, praise the Father,

praise the Son,

The son of God discloses.

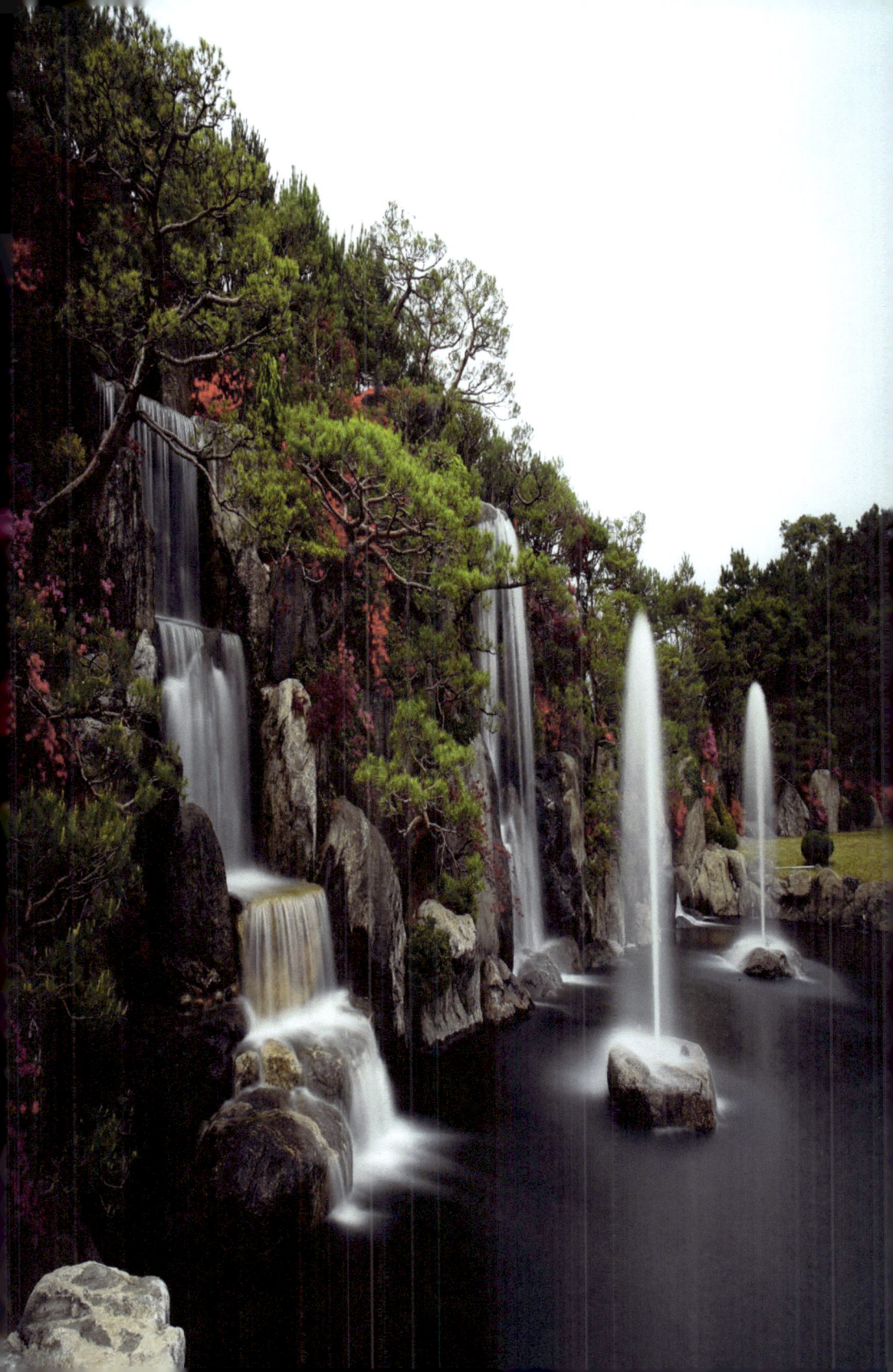

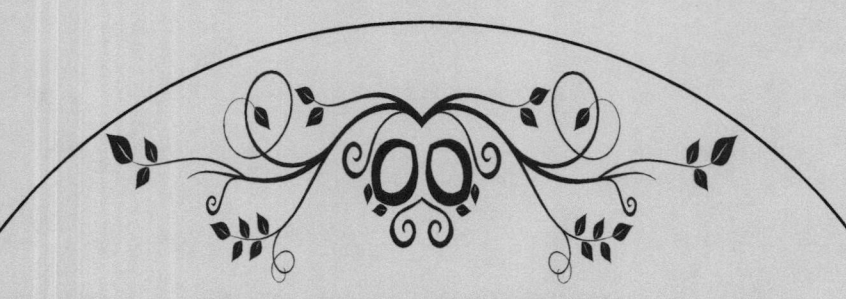

How Great Thou Art

O Lord my God,

When I in awesome wonder,

Consider all the worlds,

Thy Hands have made;

I see the stars,

I hear the rolling thunder.

Thy power throughout the –

universe displayed.

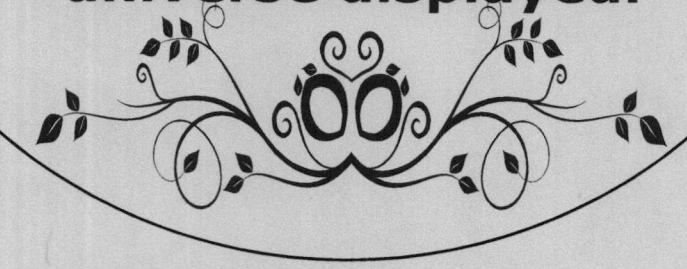

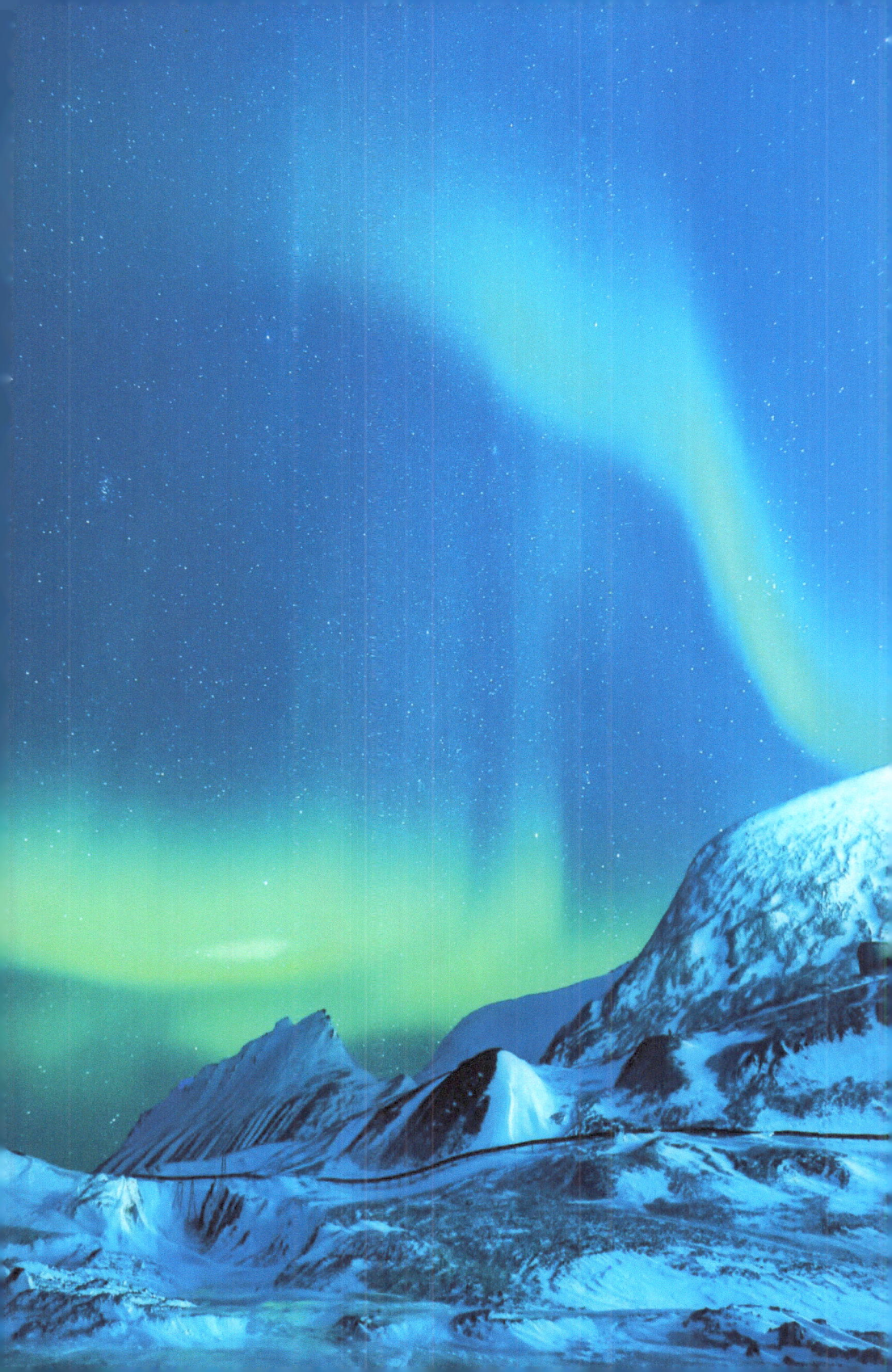

Holy, Holy, Holy

Holy, holy, holy! Lord God Almighty!

Early in the morning our song shall rise to thee,

Holy, holy, holy! Merciful and mighty,

God in three persons, blessed Trinity!"

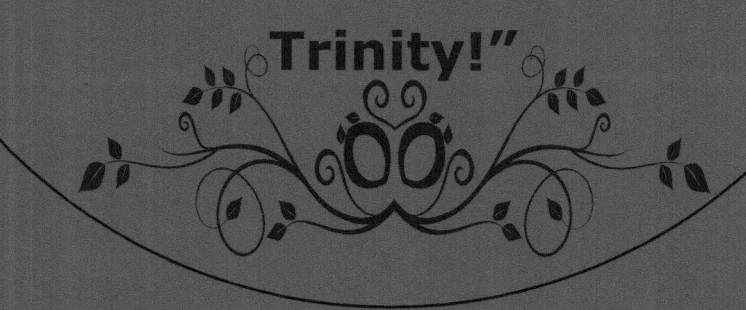

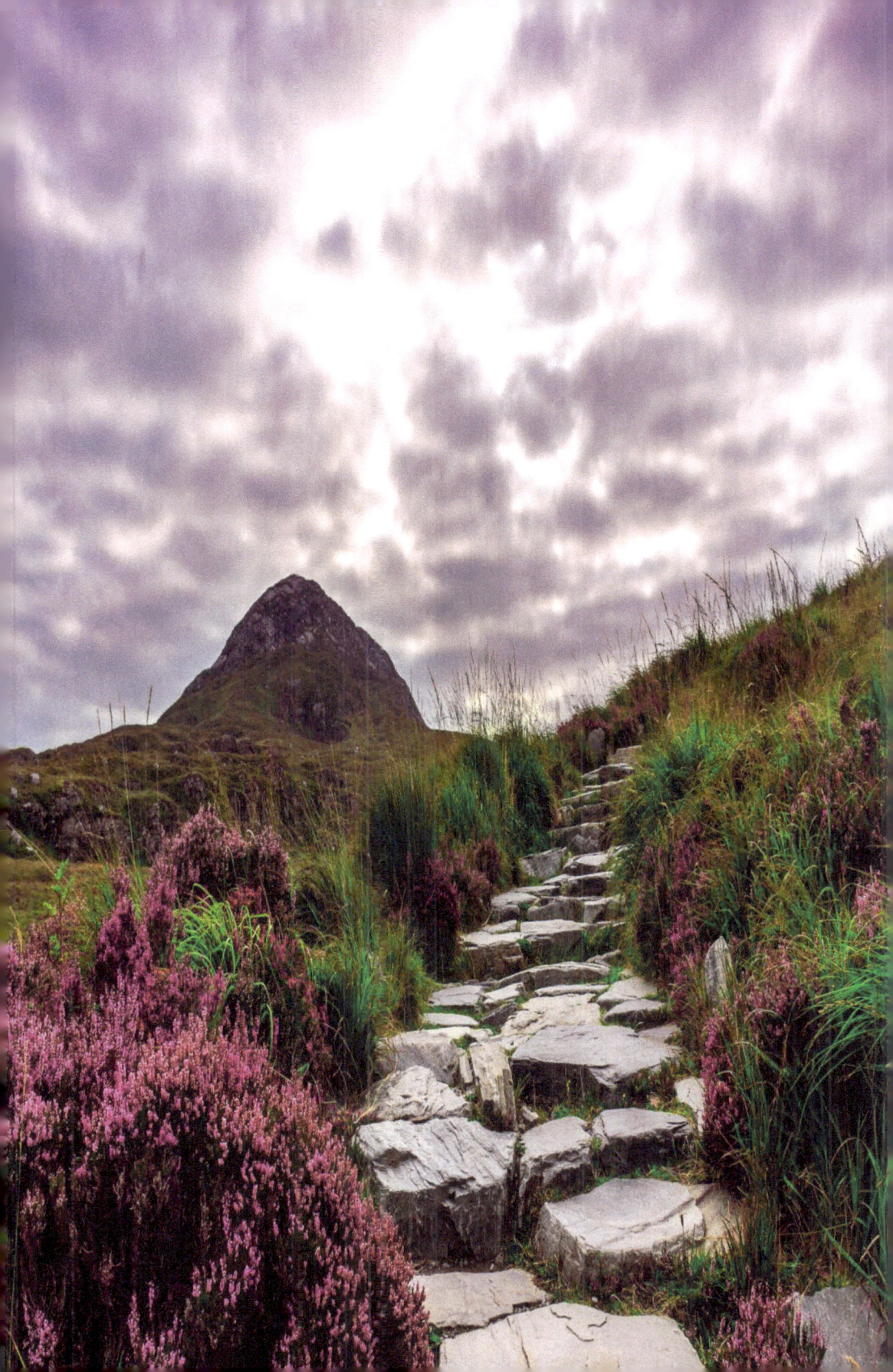

It Is Well

When peace like a river, attendeth my way;
When sorrows like sea billows roll;
Whatever my lot, Thou hast taught me to know;
It is well, it is well, with my soul.

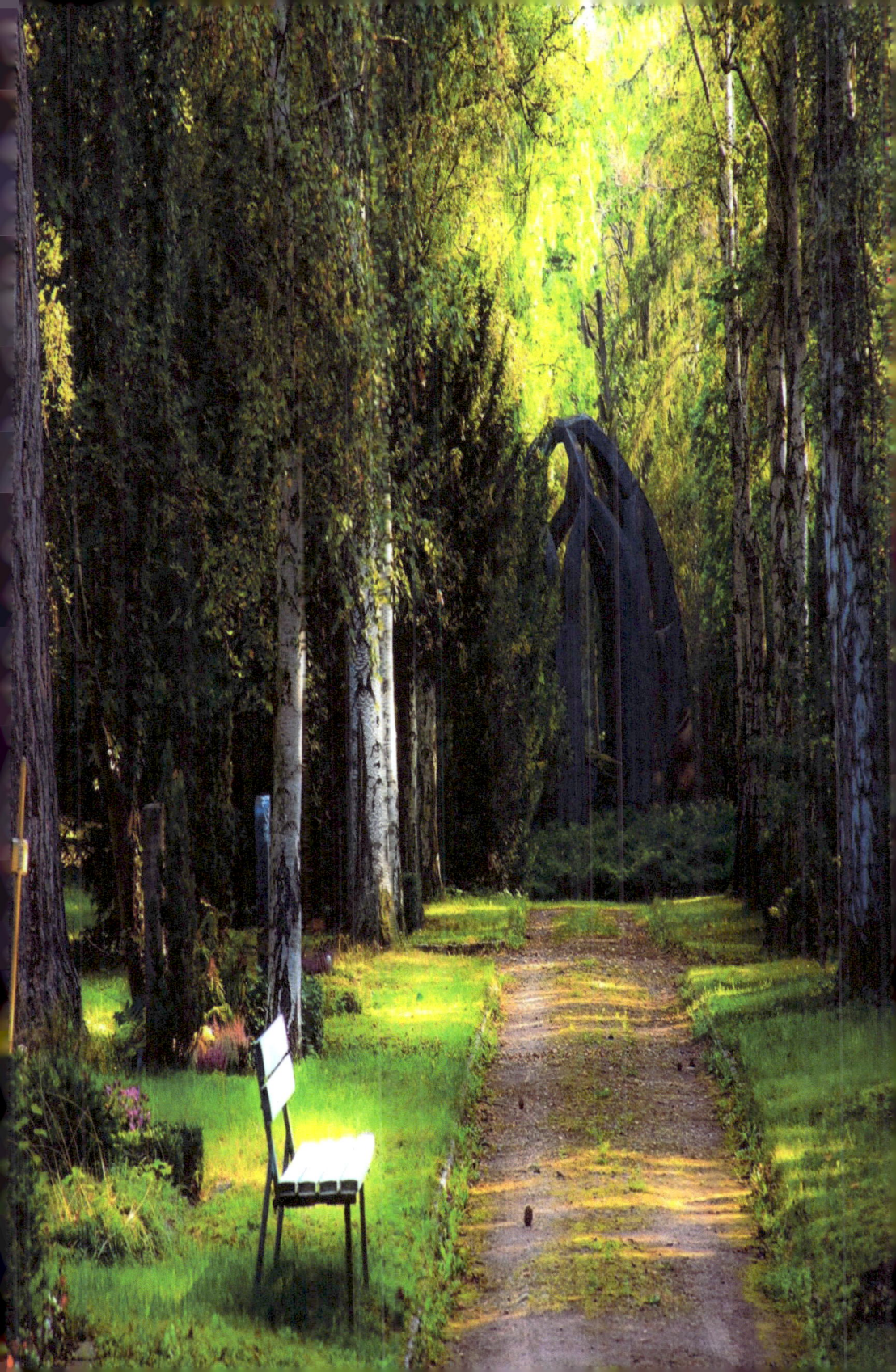

All Hail The Power of Jesus Name

All hail the power of Jesus' name!

Let angels prostrate fall,

Bring forth the royal diadem,

And crown him Lord of all.

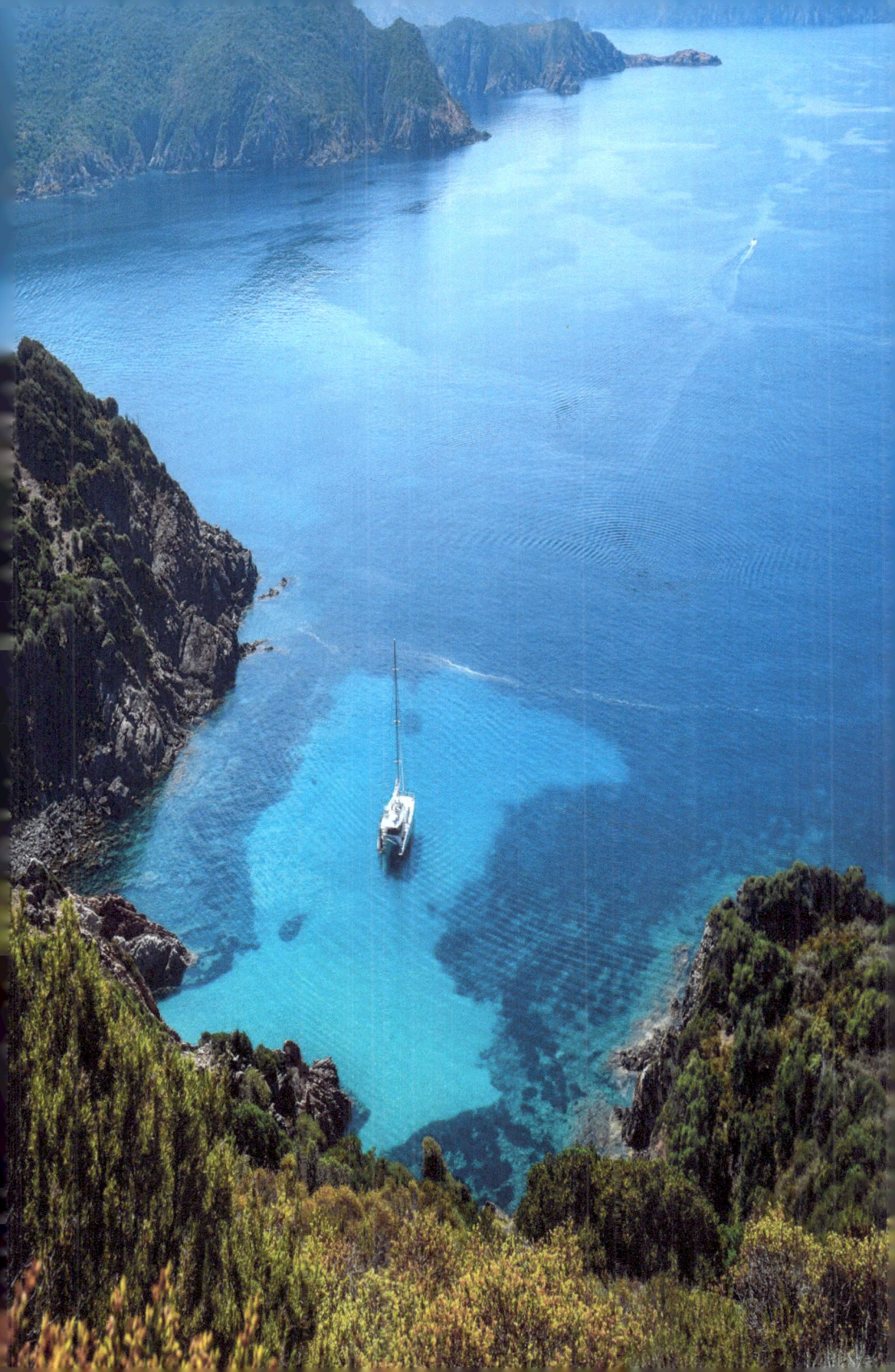

When I Survey The Wondrous Cross

When I survey the wondrous cross;

On which the Prince of glory died;

My richest gain I count but loss;

And pour contempt on all my pride.

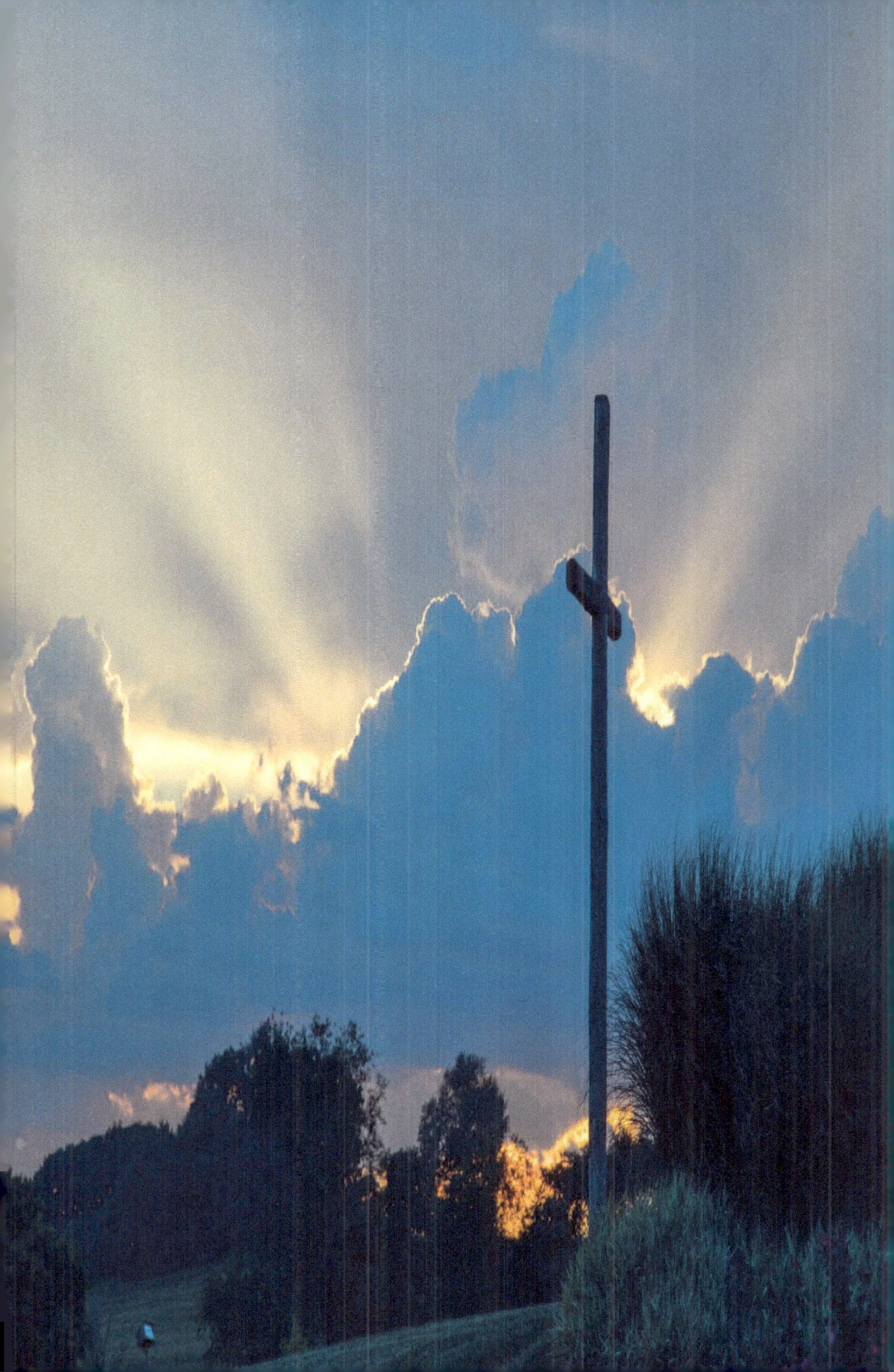

Crown Him With Many Crowns

Crown Him with many crowns,

the Lamb upon His throne;

Hark! How the heavenly

anthem drowns all music but its

own;

Awake, my soul, and sing of Him

who died for thee.

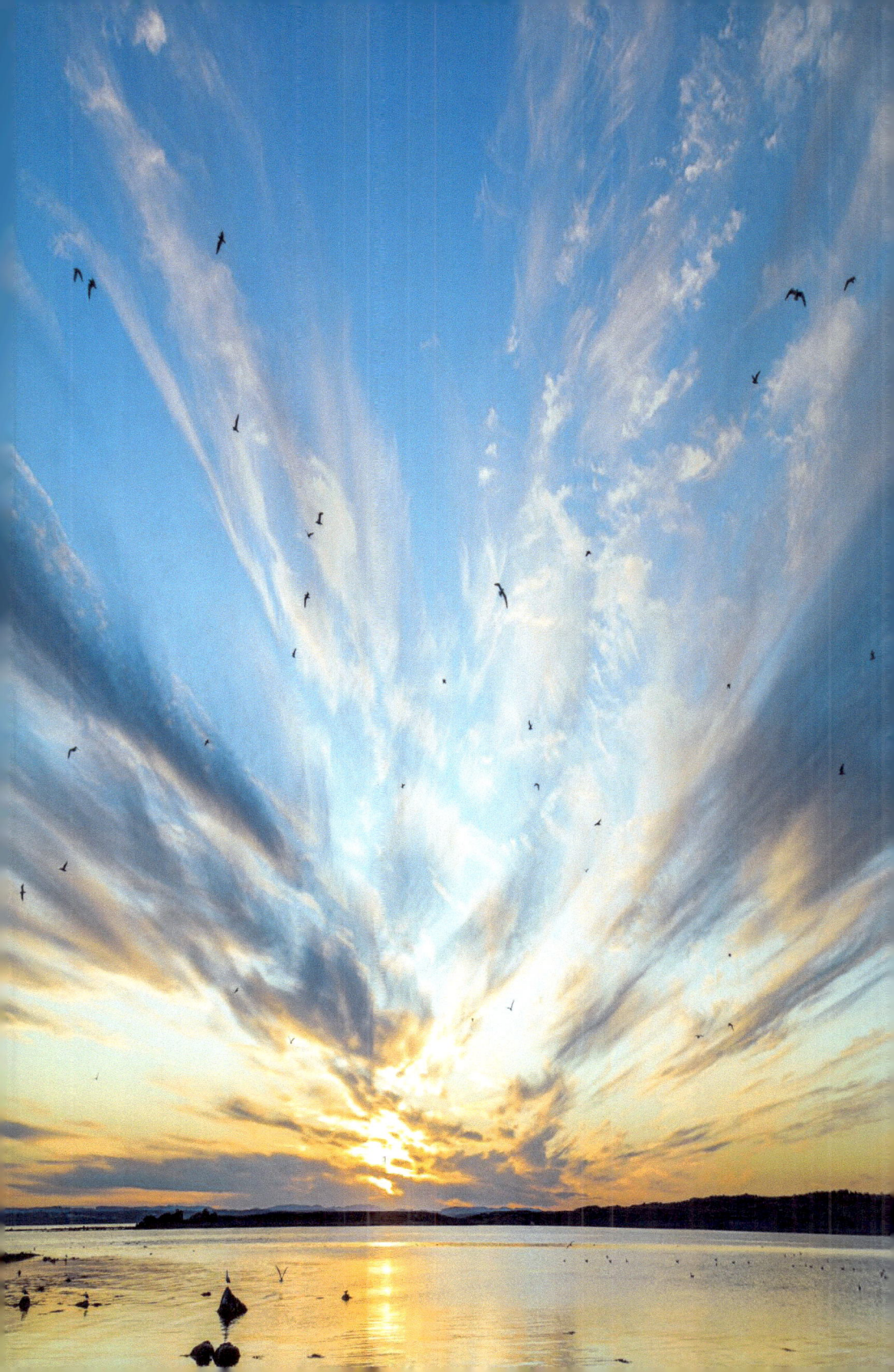

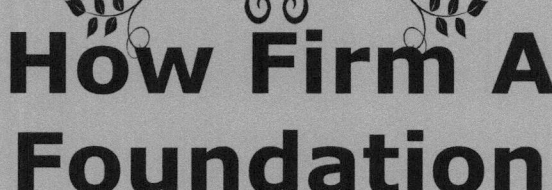

How Firm A Foundation

How firm a foundation, ye saints of the Lord;

Is laid for your faith in His excellent Word!

What more can He say than to you He hath said;

Who unto the Savior for refuge have fled?

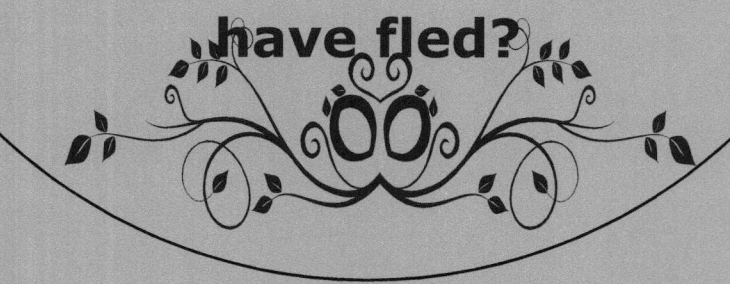

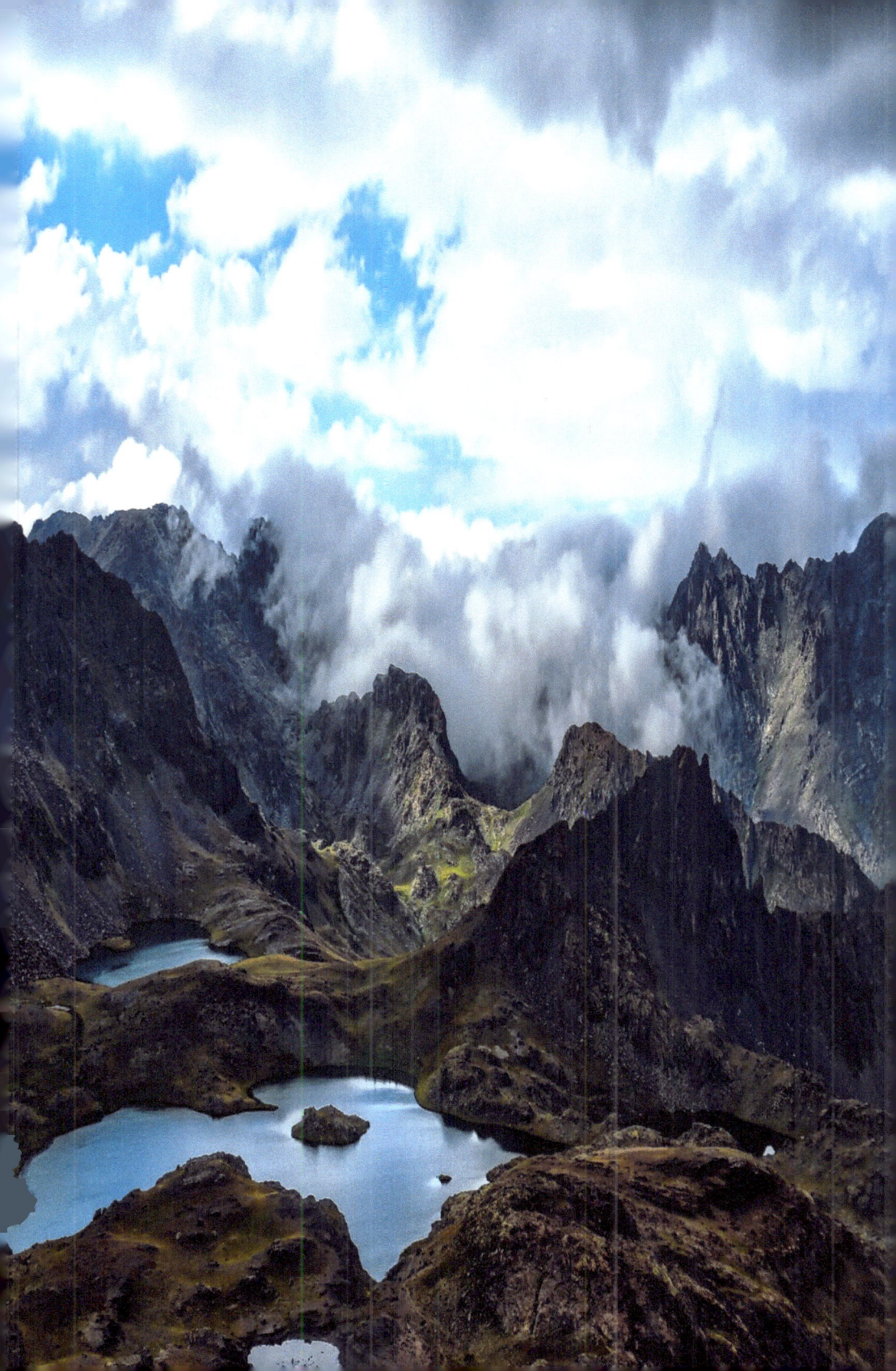

What a Friend We Have in Jesus

What a friend we have in Jesus,

all our sins and griefs to bear!

What a privilege to carry

everything to God in prayer!

O what peace we often forfeit,

O what needless pain we bear;

All because we do not carry

everything to God in prayer.

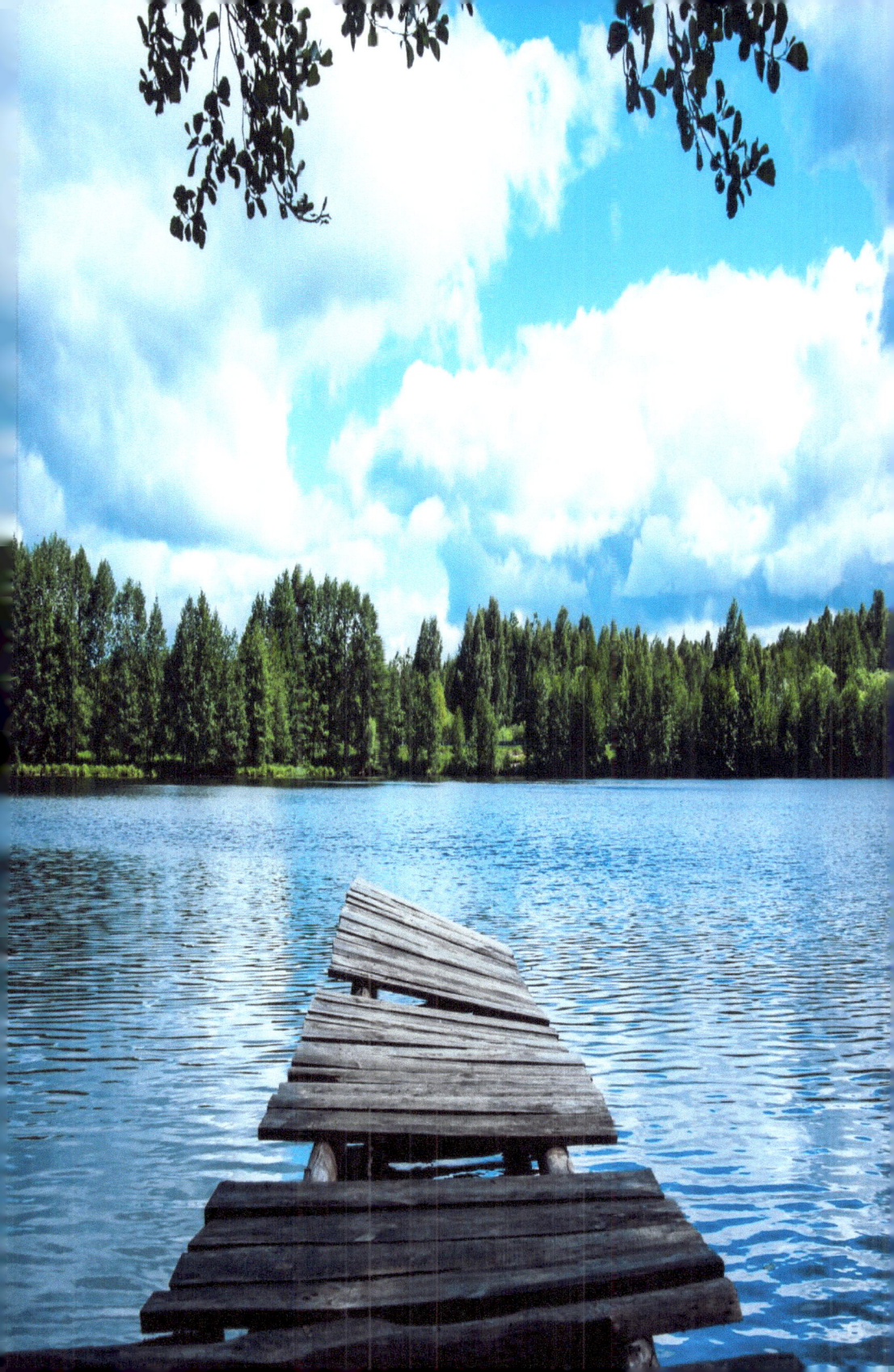

Turn Your Eyes Upon Jesus

Turn your eyes upon Jesus;

Look full in His wonderful face;

And the things of earth will

grow strangely dim;

In the light of His glory and

grace.

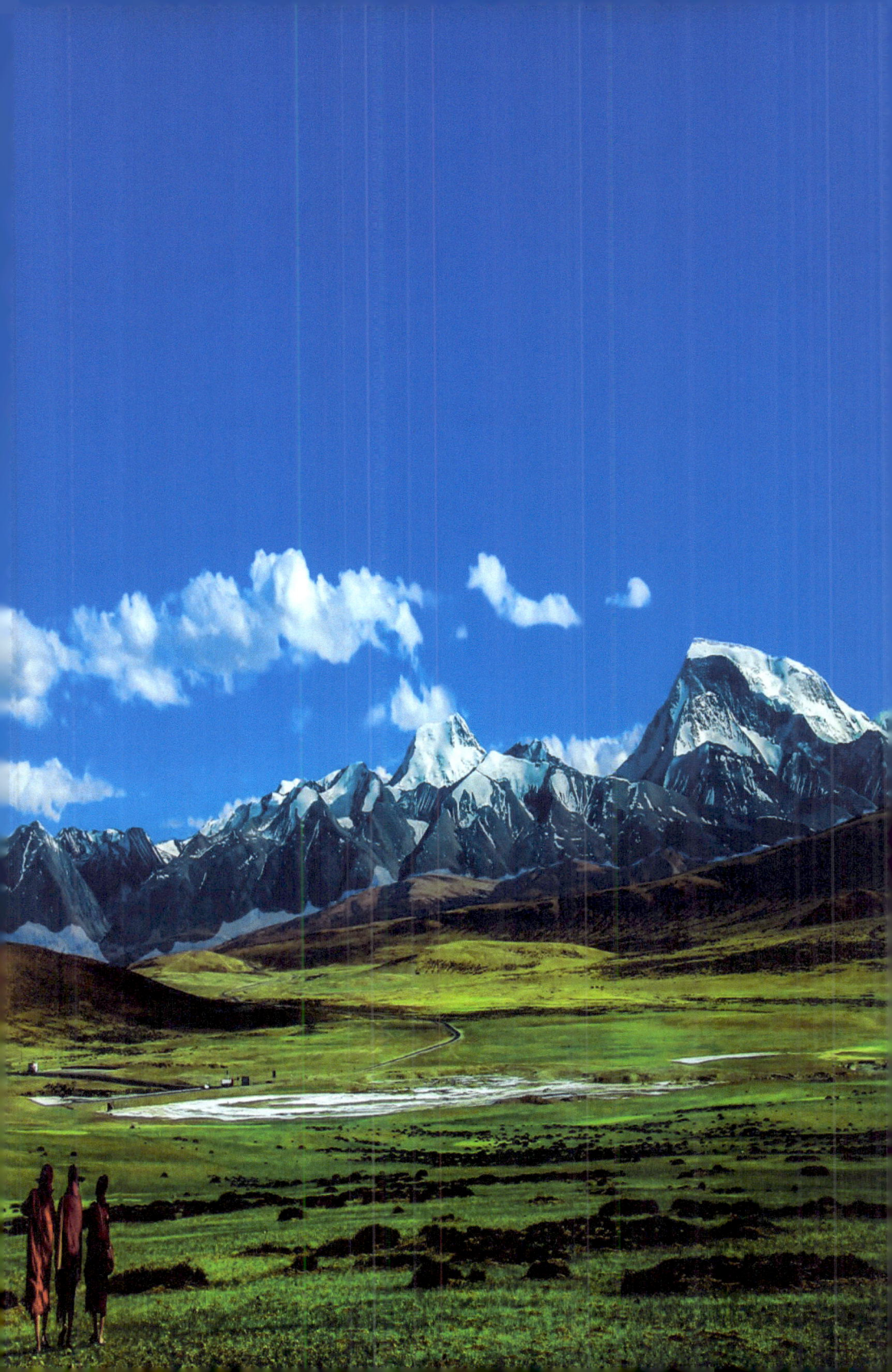

Blessed Assurance

Blessed assurance, Jesus is mine!

Oh, what a foretaste of glory divine!

Heir of salvation, purchase of God;

Born of His Spirit, washed in His blood

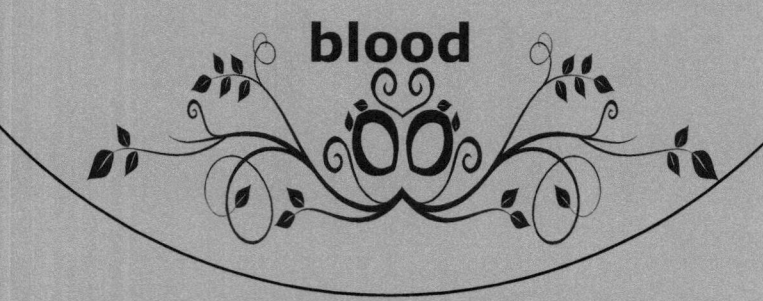

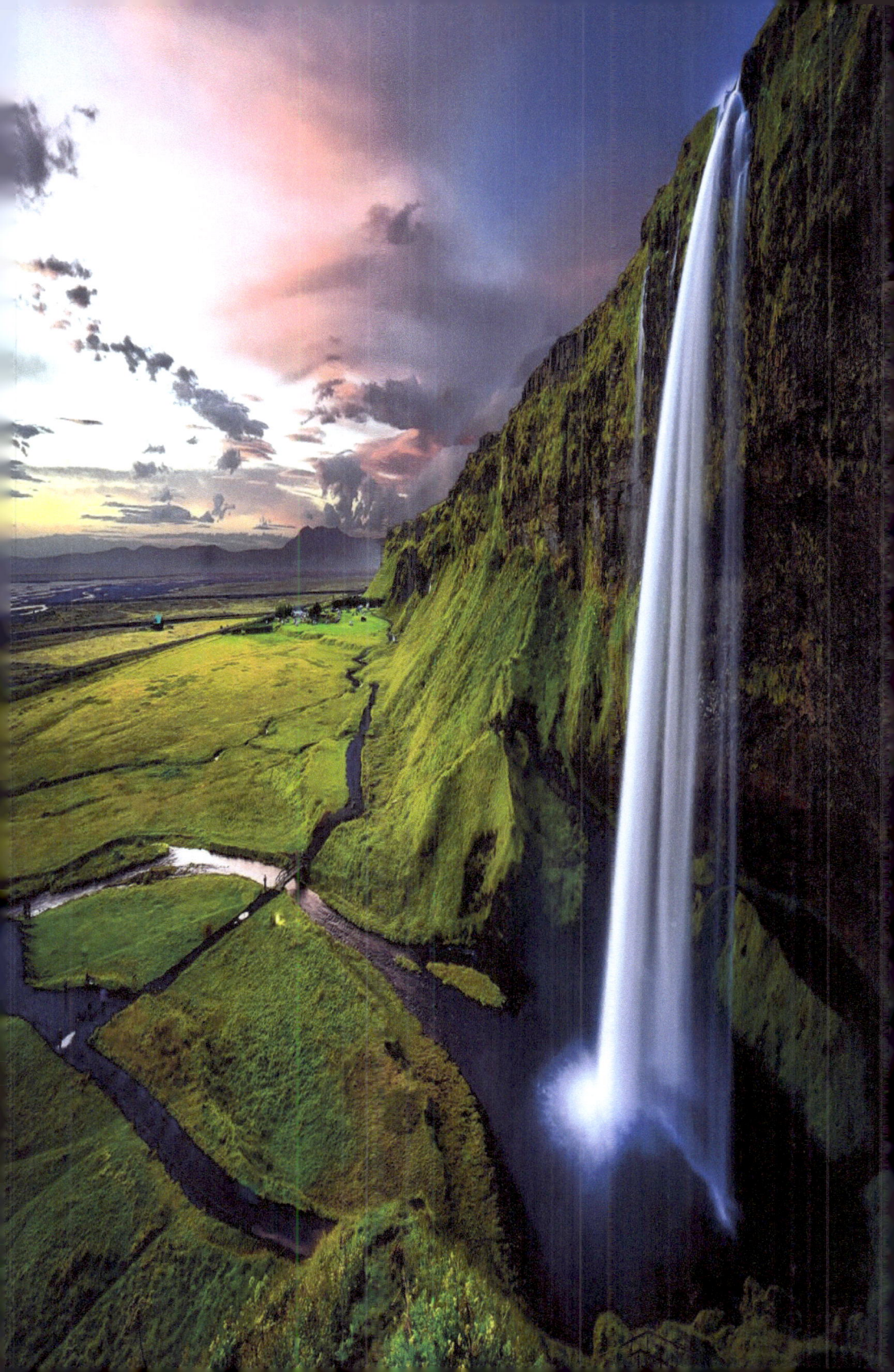

All Creatures Of our God and King

All creatures of our God and King;

Lift up your voice and with us sing;

Alleluia! Alleluia!...Praise, praise the Father, praise the Son;

And praise the Spirit, Three in One!

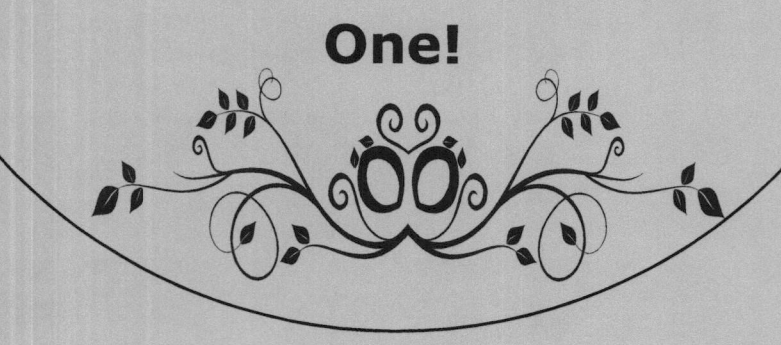

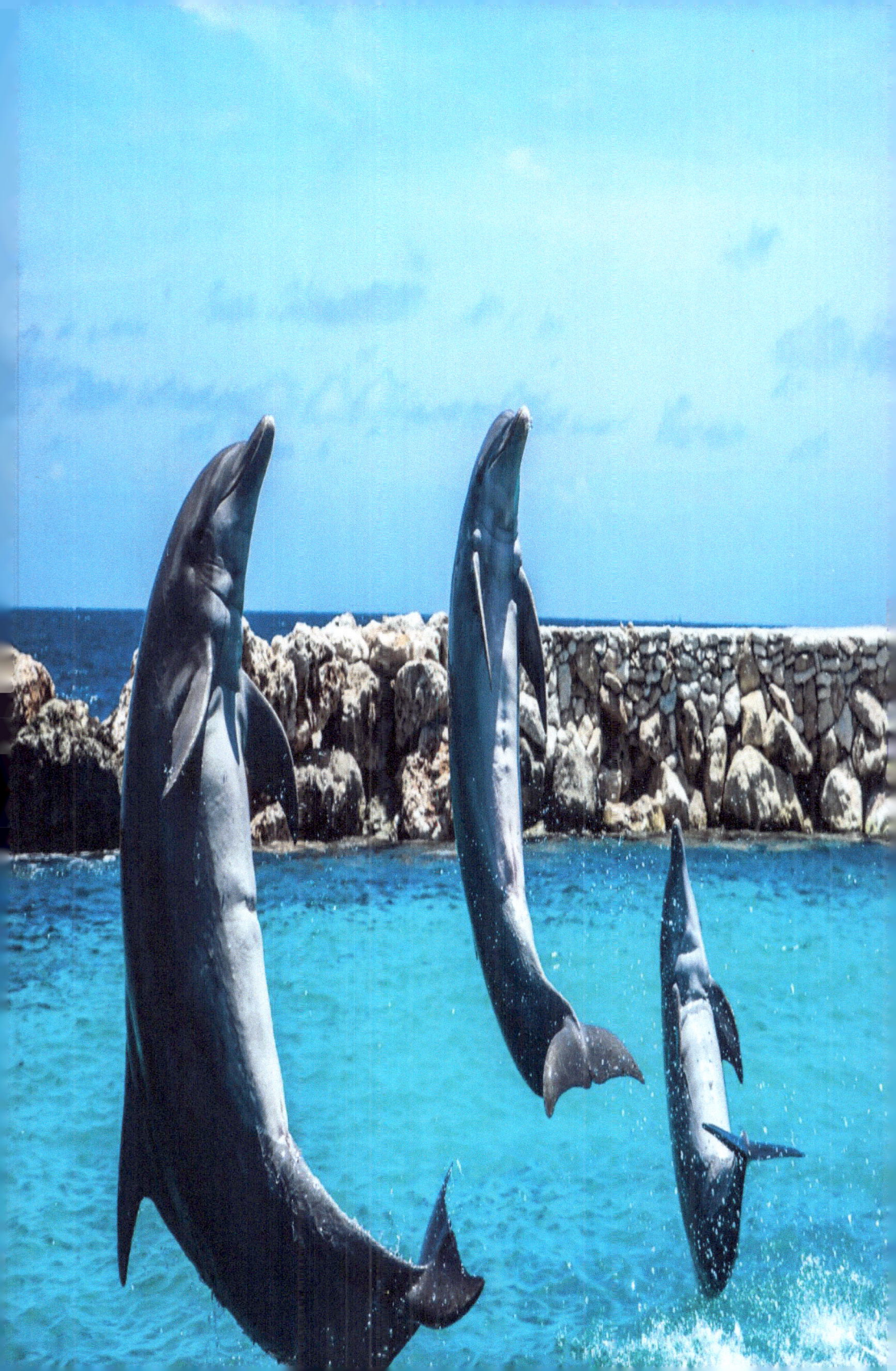

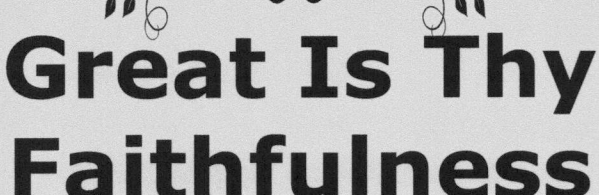

Great Is Thy Faithfulness

Great is Thy faithfulness O God my Father;

There is no shadow of turning with Thee;

Thou changest not, Thy compassions, they fail not;

As Thou hast been Thou forever wilt be.

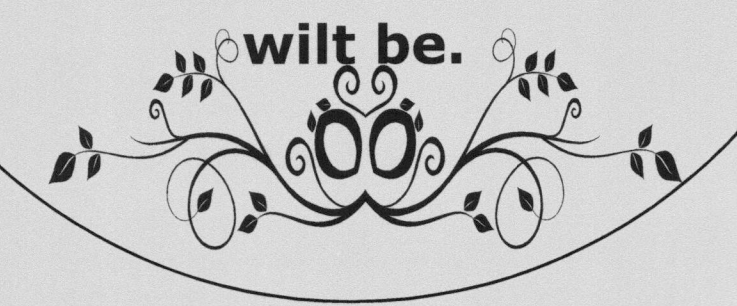

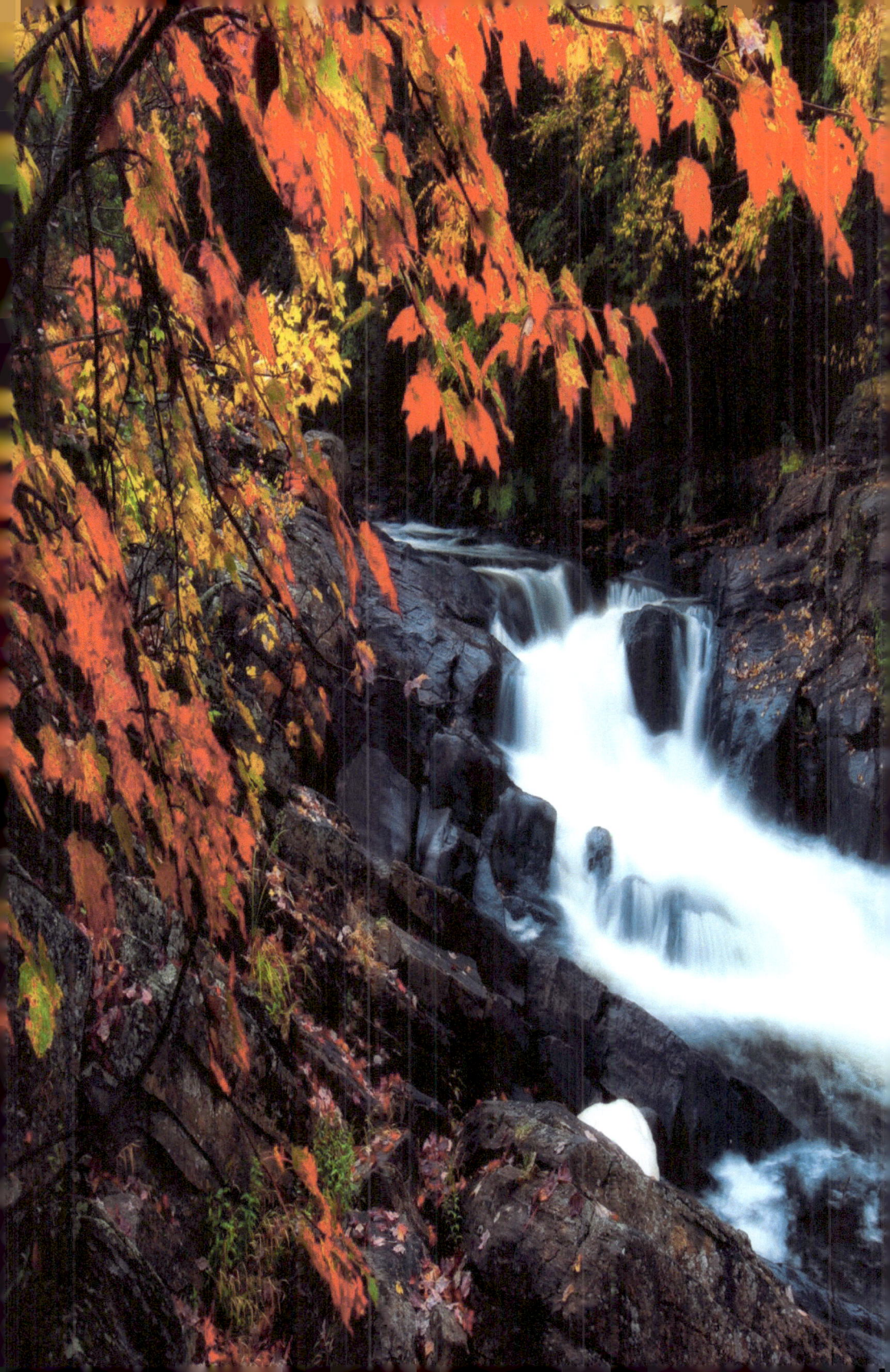

Rock Of Ages Hymn

Rock of Ages, cleft for me,

Let me hide myself in Thee;

Let the water and the blood,

From Thy wounded side which flowed,

Be of sin the double cure;

Save from wrath and make me pure.

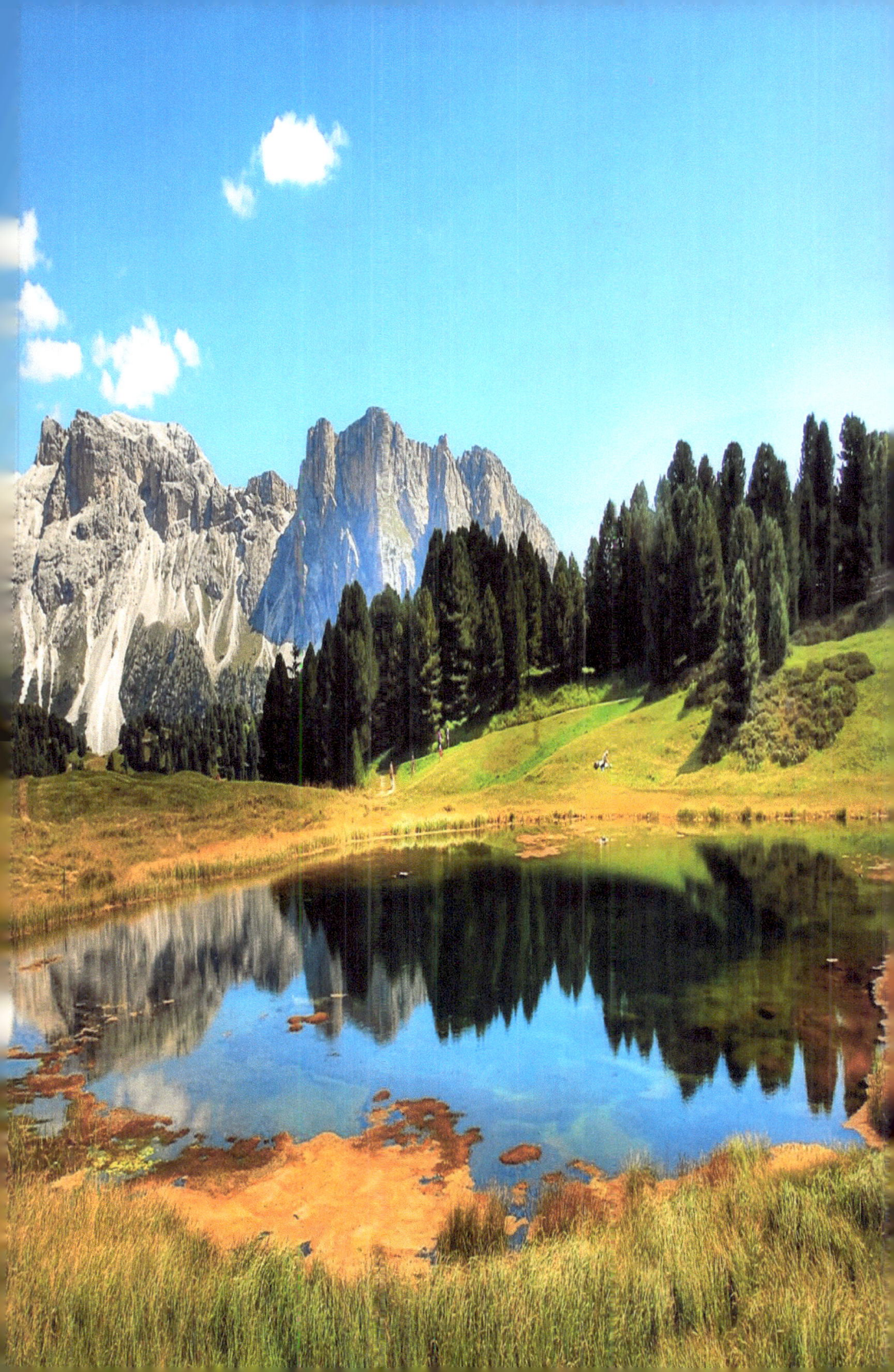

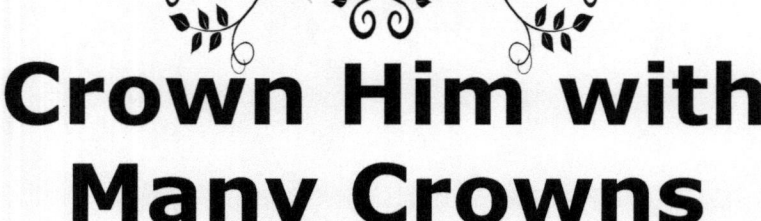

Crown Him with Many Crowns

Crown Him with many crowns,

The Lamb upon His throne;

Hark! How the heav'nly anthem

drowns

All music but its own!

Awake, my soul and sing

Of Him Who died for thee...

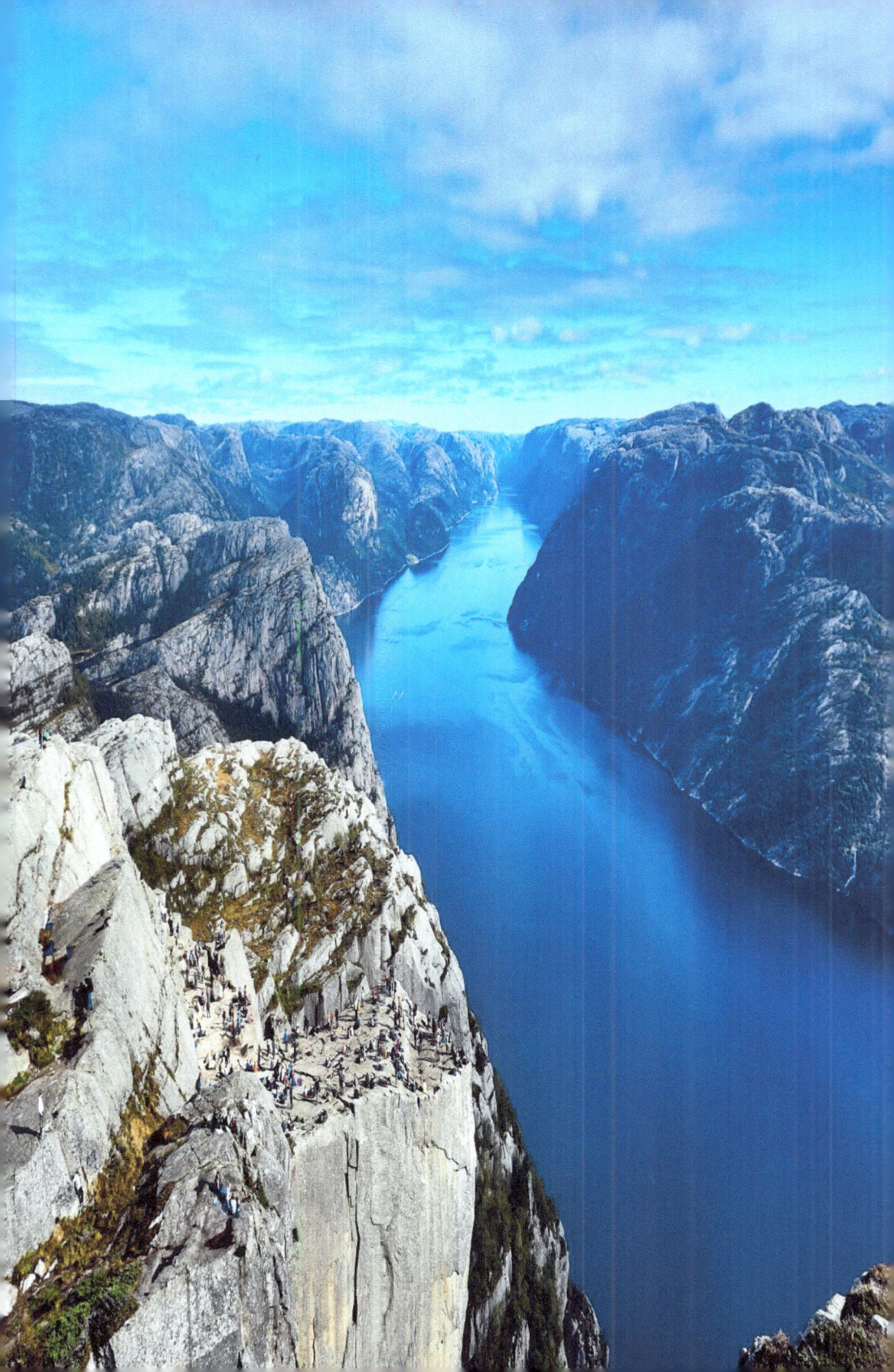

Praise To the Lord The Almighty

Praise to the Lord, the Almighty, the King of creation!

O my soul, praise Him, for He is thy health and salvation!

All ye who hear, now to His temple draw near;

Sing now in glad adoration!

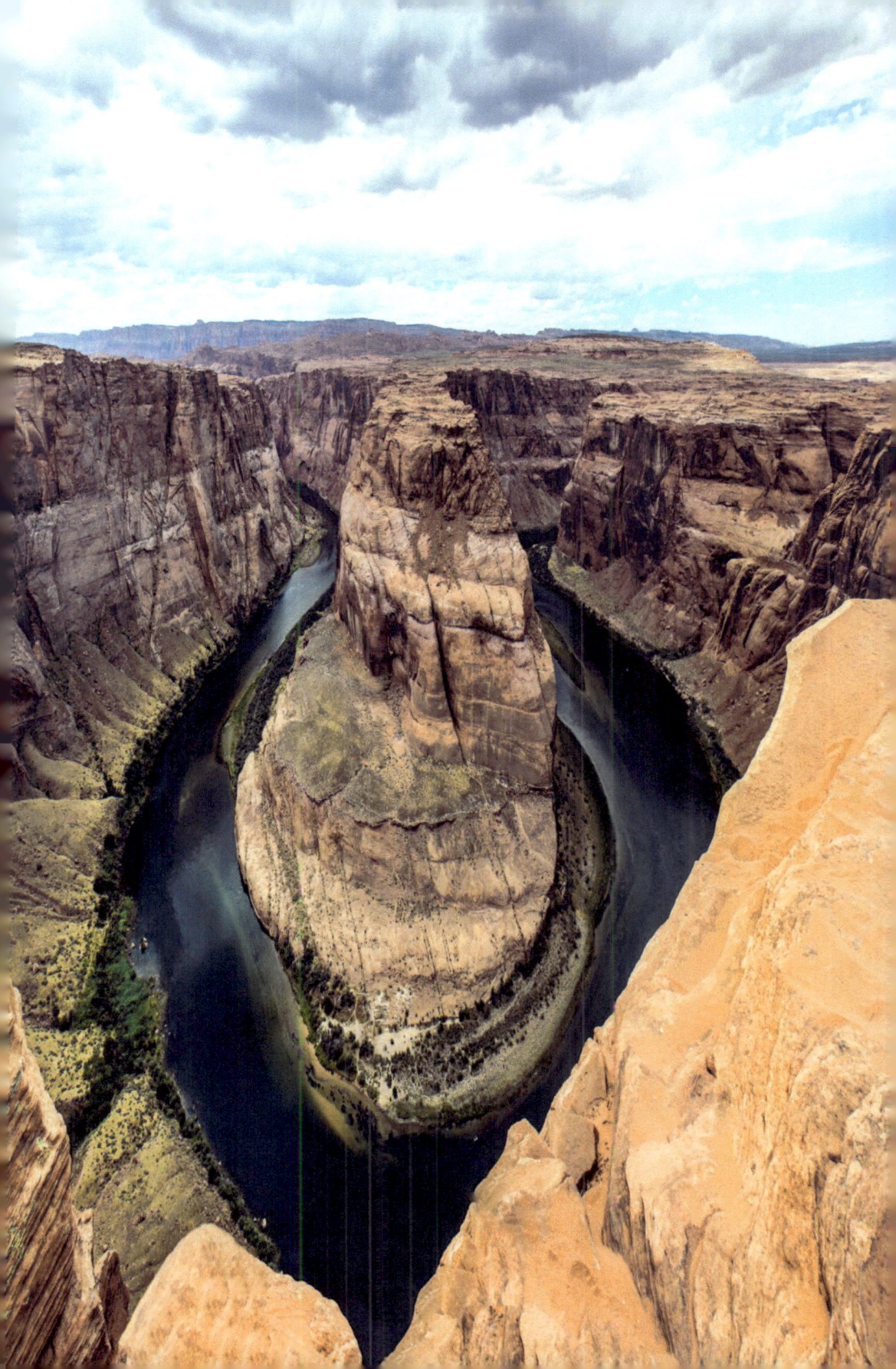

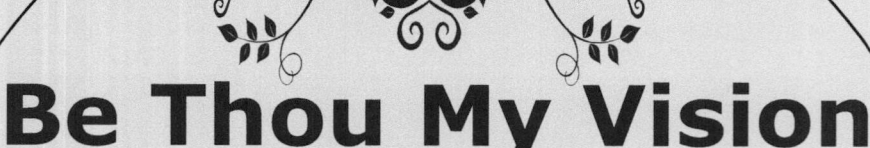

Be Thou My Vision

Be Thou my vision, O Lord of my heart;

Naught be all else to me, save that Thou art;

Thou my best thought, by day or by night;

Waking or sleeping;

Thy presence my light.

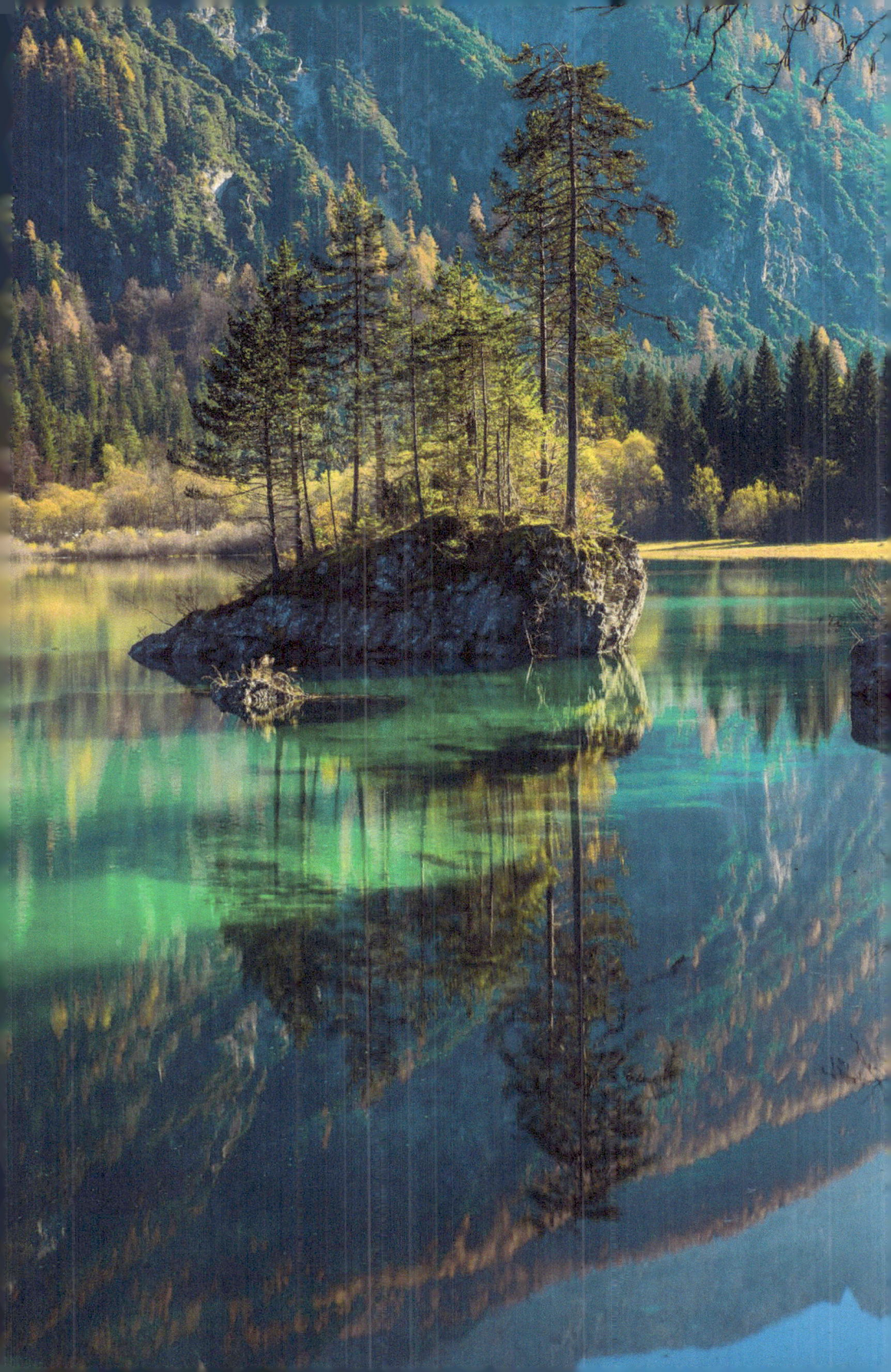

Joyful Joyful Hymn

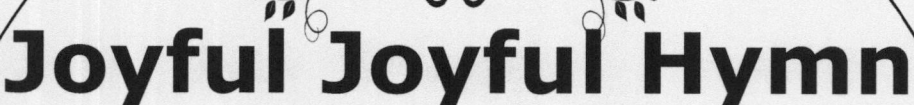

Joyful, joyful, we adore Thee,

God of glory, Lord of love;

Hearts unfold like flowers

before Thee, opening to the sun

above.

Melt the clouds of sin and

sadness;

drive the dark of doubt away;

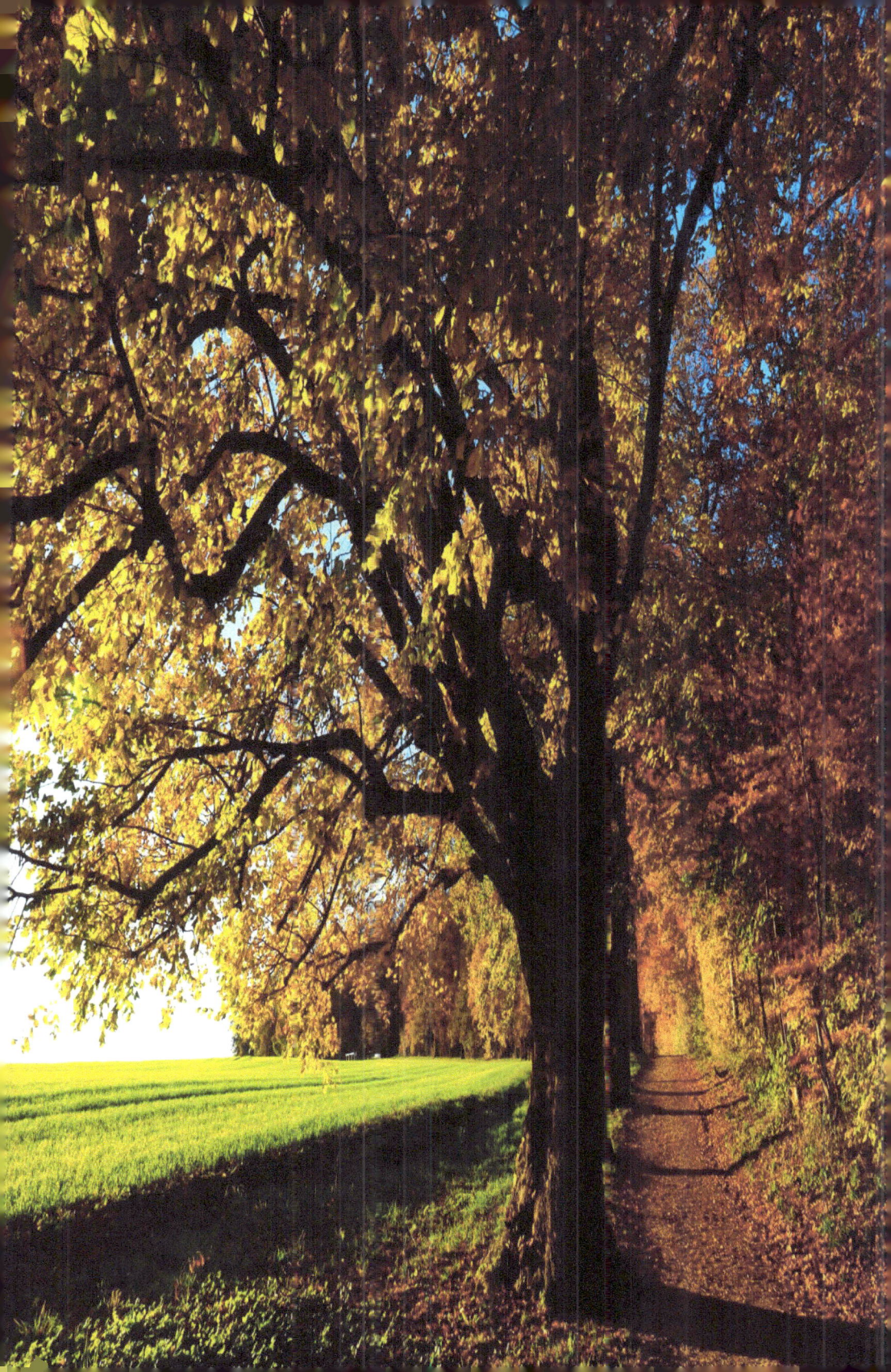

www.ingramcontent.com/pod-product-compliance
Lightning Source LLC
Chambersburg PA
CBHW040252220526
45473CB00001B/456